Essentialism

How to Feel Fulfilled from Less

Aoife Leigh Clark

DEDICATION

To Drel, always.

And to Alpha and Livie, my beloved canine companions.

CONTENTS

ACKNOWLEDGMENTS

Thanks to my darling mum, my dad, and the rest of my incredible family! As well, thank you to my readers - you keep me writing more!

INTRODUCTION

"Simplicity is complexity, resolved."
-Constantin Brancusi

What is essentialism?

Essentialism is the practice of consciously choosing less 'stuff'. It is the act of dissuading any illusions that keep us focused on the wrong things. An essence is the matter that characterizes any one thing. The essence is the indefinable quality that makes any one thing what it is; that characterizes is immortally. The essence is eternal, and wholly inalterable. All formal things are what they individually are, due to how their substance, or essence, defines them. The properties that make something what it is... to you. It's all about you, and about your embodiment of the actions that fit the life you desire to lead.

Essentially, essentialism is a paring down of the limitless options that life lies out before us. There are, quite nearly, limitless options in every which direction, regarding absolutely each and every aspect of our lives.

How do we even decide to get out of bed in the morning, once we discern the deep meaning of this simple reality? We can, literally, choose any option. There is, regardless to what you may think, absolutely nothing that can keep you from choosing what you want from the options before you. It may be hard work, and a difficult concept to grasp without complaint, but holding tight to this truth will free you. It will free you from the trappings of others' perceptions or ideas for how you should spend your time, and it will present you with adequate space within which you can curate the lifestyle you most wholeheartedly desire to lead.

How do we choose from the options? As they are limitless, we start by reexamining the most simple, basic decisions. We reassess how we are living, the habits we are embodying, and the things we are surrounding ourselves with. We go back to discerning, consciously, what the positives and negatives of each option are. We examine the trade-offs with only our truest selves in mind, to decide not only what we truly want, but what negative traits or elements we would most be able to handle. We search for the yin and yang of our optimal choosing, so that our lives are rich with fertile struggle, while also free from any unexamined elements that consistently produce byproducts that hold us back in life.

I was once living in this way, and allowed a few things to slip through the cracks, allowing for consequences that I could barely live with to seep in and take hold of my life, stopping me in my tracks; unraveling everything I had built. The clutter can really mess things up for us. As can unhappiness. Had I examined my choices in advance, and paired down the elements I was working with, I would have come upon a wisdom once it was crunch time, and I had to make the decisions I was forced into. Had I chosen a less stress-filled, overloaded existence at the time, my life wouldn't have had the opportunity to beat me up - it would never have had so much power over me! An awareness of yourself and your choices, and the positive and negatives of such, can help you lead a more pain-free, encouraging, and loving existence.

Nowadays, as I am more prepared, steadied and readied like a samurai, I do not struggle so much with decisions. Instead of hoping beyond a hope that the wind will carry my worries away and my decisions will be made for me by the world's fluctuations, I am ready for what is to come, with integrity in one hand and solace in the other. I hope for you to find this same focused simplicity in your life; and I hope that it becomes, for you, a grounding foundation that can withstand any inclimate weather to come your way.

Why Less is More

Everything doesn't matter. Absolutely everything means nothing. Nothing means anything, unless we personally undergo the process of attributing meaning to it. What happens is, once we take ownership over a person or thing, and we care about it, it can go from meaning absolutely nothing to us at all, to meaning absolutely everything in the world to us. The idea that we need certain things, or can't live without particular essentials, is blatantly untruthful. At some point in your life, most likely each and every one of those 'essentials' that you've been clinging to will end up being stripped from you, or taken away. You will eventually, more than likely, be challenged by the universe to live without each of those things, because of how it builds strength and stability of spirit, and how it teaches us more about ourselves, to try to live without whatever it is we depend on.

But why wait for the universe to decide when to challenge you? Put yourself to the test right now, by ridding your life of the various nonessentials that keep it from progressing in a wise, enlightened sense. In Buddhism, staying mindful of the world around you is of the utmost importance. This is so, in order for us to chronically discern what we feel is essential to benefitting our most pure form of existence, so that we can live our most optimally fulfilling life!

We often get motion sickness from spinning circles around ourselves, trying to taste, smell, and feel everything we get the opportunity to. The baby boomer generation really loved the idea, in my opinion, of encouraging saying 'yes' to absolutely every opportunity, in order to avoid the forsaken guilt and regret of 'not doing' or 'not trying' this thing or that thing. However, we have the power to forego this whole horrible process of missing out and regretting, simply by taking ownership over choosing what to care about, and focusing to achieve only what we feel we absolutely must. For an example, it is much easier to hike up one mountain, than three. Instead of having lifelong, never-ending to-do lists that could keep you busy for twenty lifetimes if you tried *to-do* them all, choose just a few, do them, and then choose a few more, once the time and space opens back up to you, naturally.

The idea that we can do and have it all is a delusion of the mind that prohibits us from ever seeing any true progress unfold before us. If you maximize upon what you *do* have, and what you think, say, or choose to experience, you will walk the earth a far more productive, purposeful, confident, and joyful person.

We all struggle with the 'grass is greener' syndrome of the ego, and often convince ourselves to require more than we have. Our ego makes our desires feel convincingly like necessities, tricking us into fighting for absolutely everything that comes along, rather than the select few that each individual is meant to experience and then, potentially, share in some way with the world, to better both ourselves and the world surrounding. We always want what we can't have, and this mindset will always get in the way of our getting what we want, regardless of how we like to think it'll just work out magically for us. Let me tell you, I've tried every kind of magic and magick out there, and none of it can help you forego having to do the work yourself, of streamlining and cementing your desires into your foundational being.

We are so easily stretched far too thin in this world of excess. Waste piles up into walls that keep us bound to our place. Much like ruffling through a pile of garbage, we quickly sort and discern from the limitless options around us, oftentimes choosing whatever is most handy or accessible; oftentimes, choosing the simple path of least resistance. I know more than most, as I used to be deathly frightened of confrontation, or others trying to 'figure me out'. I didn't want anyone to know that I was too busy to choose consciously. I didn't want, in fact, to be 'found out' for my negligence of, and ignorance to, the options before me. Like a child cheating on an exam, I wanted to get away with my ignorance, and not have to do the necessary work to research and prepare for what was to come. Hell, I still struggle with this on a regular basis, as most of us do. I struggle with truly living up to my ideal self without allowing my ego to take the ideals I honor and twist them toward my manipulative, selfish benefit. It's a hard thing to do. However, by pairing your focus down to a few distinct areas of personal importance, it will all be a whole hell of a lot easier, to be sure! Conflicts *will* occur in your life, whether you like it or not - will you be ready?

As many qualms as I may have with the education system as a whole, there are some gems that still ring true. The idea of needing to research, study and prepare is very useful to all of life. And pop-up quizzes? Horrible - absolutely horrible - but genius. Absolutely, we need to be ready for what we don't expect. And this can, indeed, be one of the most flabbergasting ideas. You wonder to yourself, 'Where on Earth do I begin?' when looking into the abyss of opportunity and choice. You convince yourself that it's too much work, too much to ask of yourself, and that you don't really need to do it. You tell yourself you're going places, and talk yourself into the idea that compared to the rest of the world, you're doing quite well, if you're being honest with yourself. Bullocks. This is mental clutter at its most successful; its most callous. And this clutter is garbage.

Successful and honorable individuals do not delude themselves into thinking that, by comparing themselves on a curve to the rest of the world, they are off the hook in regards to having to work hard on bettering their behaviors. They choose *not* to sink into the illusion that, just because the world has bigger problems than them, this means they don't need to try. Rather, they see those big world problems, and they realize that, by relinquishing their ego and empowering their choices, they benefit the rest of the world. They recognize how they truly make an impact. They see just how foolish it is for anyone to excuse themselves from the self-work, for any reason. They see clearly the ultimate truth that we all affect one another in ways that may seem too subtle and unperceivable to the ignorant eye. And, what's more, they live their life through the integrity of the choices they make; by which I mean, they think of the world in a broad view, with the understanding that we all have a higher purpose of contribution to offer the world, and that we choose whether or not we follow the enlightened path with every choice we make.

By discerning what is absolutely essential to our existence, and then eliminating every non-essential, we gain the insight; the clarity into who we are, what we hold true to, and, essentially, what defines us. Choosing to focus more on less elements will give your life a focused meaning and purpose to carry you through your existence. You don't want to end up trapped in a web of your own messied attempts at purposeful action. You want to be supported by a tightly woven, creatively designed hammock. And hopefully, on a beach, in the sun, without the sunburn.

MIN & MAX

Maximalists

I used to embody the very idea of a maximalist. In college and just after, was when I excelled the most in my maximalism. I was attending multiple colleges at once, as I toggled between four differing degree tracks (thank goodness they overlapped some, or else I would really have gone nuts). I was, quite literally, trying to do everything. I wanted to absorb and get as much out of the college experience as I possibly could. Maximalists live in excess, as was I, in taking on more than my fair share of classes and majors. Maximizers abide by the 'more is more' way of viewing the world, rather than the minimalist 'less is more' perspective.

There is definitely something to exploring maximalist perspectives, however, and I honestly urge you to get a little crazy, if you never have before. It's super fun to slurp up the world around you whole, just as it's exciting to eat a whole carton of your favorite ice cream in one sitting, but these actions are not sustainable, and they detract from the whole; they weaken and lay ruin to the greater good. I mean, just look at climate change, garbage islands, and the way consumable meat is raised.

We have been living in excess for a very long time now, and our earth is hurting, as a result. We need to keep to our own more often than we do, to help the earth sustain herself. However, this doesn't mean you have to abstain from adventure! Not in the least! Explore the earth, and sip from her nectar! Just, be sure you don't guzzle it all up, so that there's none left to share with those around you. We are stronger as a whole; and, therefore, we protect our own, and help to sustain the masses, rather than just preserving our selves.

Multitasking is a gross illusion we delude ourselves into thinking proves positive results. There is a firm delineation that must be made here. We can improve and speed our habits in positive ways through multitasking by, say, doing our laundry while reading a book, or folding socks while listening to music; but, burnout is sure to occur if you're attempting the kind of multitasking that requires your awareness and attention to split. Especially avoid this while learning new skills! Trust me, the girl who went to so many colleges that she confuses them and what they were for.

Once your attention and awareness are split, all of your abilities split. It's not like our brain suddenly doubles in capacity. No. You are absorbing half as much of whatever you split your attention between. Whether it's hanging out with your children while working, or texting while driving, or cooking while cleaning. Your brain literally splits its attention, and, like a pie chart, your abilities are split: you are half as good at everything you combine when multitasking. Further, it has been proven to actually slow us down, when we multitask compared to when we focus on one task at a time. Scientifically, this has been quantified: multitasking is not nearly as efficient or productive as we would like to believe. It may be more fun, and elapse boredom more fluently, but it is counterproductive and does waste time and effort. Focus is key.

Minimalists

In these ideas of essentialism and minimalism, the focus is on only a few things, rather than the many. The focus is on cherishing and emulsifying with everything you hold dear, rather than trying to quickly slurp up everything in sight. This is a disciplined pursuit of much, much less. Instead of pouring your efforts out to everything that attracts itself to you, you choose what to accept in joy, and what to turn away in grace. You will go from spending your time and energy up to the brim, without any left for yourself, no focus in sight, and no real, true, attainable goals on the horizon; to, wisely investing your time and energy effectively, to get as much as you can out of each thing you engage with. You will treasure, and hold sacred, the things that matter to you. You will reap more benefits than you can imagine - you will feel more deeply, have more meaningful interactions, you will lose the anxiety and the fear that plague your life, and you will be free; you will feel free. By choosing to focus on less now, you will receive more later. You will be capable of producing and offering your best opinion, in your highest form, to the world. When you are concise and clear with your intentions and embodiments, the world responds more clearly and with precision.

There exists a particular triviality of nonsense that wastes our time and energy like mad; it drains us of the energy it takes to live a fully embodied, pure life. From television, to facebook, video games, Instagram, twitter, tinder, and all the other online worlds that exists out there in the inter-webs, these are all distractions, and they may be distracting us from the very vital essentials we absolutely need to be happy, and to survive. You may have been soul-sucked into Twitterland, too preoccupied to hear for what your heart is truly, deeply longing. If you take but a momentary lapse, you may be able to hear it calling out. In the world today, you almost have to make yourself uncomfortable - force yourself to feel a little bad - in order to want to change, and hear the winds blow so you know which way to go.

There are definite perks to being available less often, and to limiting your usability and visibility. By deciding not to post every photo your family takes online for all the world to see, and not always texting everyone back immediately, you can establish boundaries for yourself, that will effectively free up a lot of your emotional clouding, thus freeing up your energy to explore more of the things that will make you happier. You know, I'm not dissing on having a lot of people in your life. That's awesome, and a gift, if you've got it. Don't shut the people you love out. But do choose to be less available, at least just for a little while, to see if this makes an impact.

As you begin to minimize your focus, you will encounter differing views on how to go about this, from an essentialist perspective. Some would suggest hacking away at the nonessential elements you witness in your life, as though it's a fight you must struggle through daily to win. I don't fully understand or agree with this sentiment. I feel that, once you know what you do not want, and are focused on what you do, allow a simple ritual of maintenance, in giving the ideas, adventures, and goals back to the universe, for somebody else to embody and grow inspired by. Just as energy healers give unnecessary energies back to the universe in order to clear out energy blockages, you will simply no longer give energy or attention to those things that do not align with or serve your higher purpose. In other words, I choose not to see this process as so aggressive, and choose, instead, to perceive it as effortless maintenance. If you give any thing too much negative, or aggressive / defensive energy, you then attract more negative energy towards you. What you output, you get back in three. And sticking with minimalists, is the way to be.

Balance

Every single time that you get duped into thinking that something has a hold on you, look down at your hands. I guarantee you that you will find that you are, in fact, the one with the stronghold on the things that keep you. We truly are our own worst enemies. We want to multitask because it's more fun, even if it isn't more efficient; we want to let others take the brunt of our fall, and help us clean up our messes, as though it is their civic duty; we want to cheat the systems in our favor, because we feel the world owes us, or has dealt us a poor hand; and we want to take everything we can while we go down in flames. But we do not have to. We don't have to 'perish like a fading horse', slurping up all we can and then burning out before we've experienced the full spectrum of what life offers. We can narrow. We can choose, consciously, from the spectrum, to carefully balance out our life. However, we don't want to narrow ourselves too much, either. To every yin, there is a yang. And that is what we are searching for: the ever-revolving balance between our yin and yang energies, that supports and nourishes us to be all that we can; contribute all that we can.

You can, then, apply this idea of balance to every aspect of your life. From the things that you own to the way that you utilize your space; from your mindset to how you disperse your time and energy.

The Utility of the Item

Utilitarianism and essentialism go hand in hand, to an extent, as utilitarianism focuses upon the utility, or functionality of an item, and essentialism focuses on an item's essence, or defining quality. One is more practical and impersonal of a mindset; the other more emotional, and personal. While using utilitarianism to focus upon an object's usability, you can add an essence of essentialist thinking in the mix, to see how it impacts you, on a personal level. In my book on decluttering, I advise how one should never keep any object one does not love. If it doesn't bring joy to you, throw it out! What you love, cherish.

What you use for utility can be narrowed down to the things you do have, rather than things you think you need. You can choose to expect more from each item in your life. Have each item do more, and play a wider range of roles in your life; a wider range of function. Expect unexpected functions from the items you have. Not in a way that is dangerous at all; just, in a way that maximizes the utility of the object, so that you have no need for excess items. For example, use a spoon to peel your apples and to juice your lemons and limes - it works wonders; you truly do not need peelers or juicers for that level of interaction. There is, also, a lot of functional furniture and house planning research out there, to support utility in your home. Murphy Beds, for example, are a super-chic, modern version of the old drop-down bed. Murphy beds turn into coffee tables, desks, or various other spatial outlays. There is, now, so much furniture that adjusts within your space, that you could really maximize on any minimal amount of space, which is especially helpful if you have a big family, or a small living space. Further, an effective way of both avoiding clutter and maximizing space, is to ensure that every object you love, keep, and enjoy has its very own, designated space wherein which to thrive, and dissuade clutter away.

The characteristics of choosing to fix rather than throw away an object or item are of much interest to me. I find that, our chronic tendencies to either horde or discard every object in sight, are both equally unhealthy. They are both symptoms of a greater dis-ease: an inability to acutely discern what it is you really want. If you choose to research and fix some of the things you automatically turn to throw away, you may get to keep a particular treasured item longer, or continue to use something that you thought was a goner. You may be able to find some super fun, versatile, and ingenious ways of utilizing the oddest of things! Just search for the Buzzfeed article on pool noodles and their versatility; I promise you will not be disappointed with all the ways they come up with utilizing pool noodles outside their function.

Now, this idea that what you choose to use for utility can be narrowed down to what you already have, can be readily applied to your personal, emotional, and proficient capacities. Rather than focusing on how you don't know how to do this or that, attack a problem from an angle that you *are* familiar with. Get creative in how you address and assess the problems or roadblocks in your path, and then face them, and handle them with integrity and strength, doing the best you can, instead of trying to skirt around them unnoticed, or solve them in ways that dishonor your true essence.

This goes for food as well. Don't go to the grocery store only once a month to stock up - you are sure to waste, unless you're some sort of food planning expert (in which case, more power to you!). Try to get creative in the kitchen, rather than buying groceries for recipes and accidentally wasting what the recipe doesn't call for, because you have no idea what to do with the items you bought outside of the recipe. Try to live off of just the essentials for a little while, to push your creativity cooking juices to flow! This tactic of shopping only for essentials will help your mind, your fridge, and your wallet!

BURNOUT

The pressure to try everything

Others' expectations can freeze us in our place. I have struggled somewhat, as most Americans have, in the areas of mental illness, and suspect that much of it, for many of us, is onset by our struggle with attempting to be something for somebody else. Whether, in your case, it's that you want to be everything to everyone in your life; or that you feel the pressure to appease your elders or peers; or, that you set nearly unreachable goals for yourself and compare every success to this idealized foil characteristic of your true self... Like a reflection that ruins you. You need to choose the elements of your life for *you,* and not for anybody else.

As a tangent: I struggled greatly in separating myself from my parents' expectations of whom I should be. When I had moved away for the first time, I struggled to see why I even mattered at all, after I separated myself from their opinions... I figured, if I wasn't making them happier with my successes, I was an immediate failure, and was overwhelmed with disappointment: from my perceived image of my folks' disappointment, to my perception of my own failure, and the disappointment that stemmed from this as a result. But the crazy, crazy thing is: I did it all to myself. Once I freed myself from my own mental constraints, and I truly stopped living for their expectations, nothing bad happened, and they moved on with their lives. As it turned out, they had only been waiting for me to stop needing their advice all the time, to stop soliciting it. And they didn't solely place their happiness in my successes, as I had presumed! I tortured myself to make my parents happier, when they were just happy so long as I was happy. Once I decided to make myself happy - I mean, *truly* happy - the rules shifted; the game changed, and all of this beautiful space opened up in my life, for me to then choose how to fill. This is when I truly curated my life.

Don't let others decide how you live your life. This statement doesn't have to be dramatic or difficult - it is the essentiality of all essentialism. You deserve to decide for yourself, simply because you are human. It is an instinctual, essential, given truth to our existence. As the gorgeously under-rated, world-changing feminist musician Ani DiFranco so eloquently said, "your body is your only true dominion". This is it. She captured it. And thus, you should feel confident and content in the idea that your body, your mind, your soul, and your choices, are all your own.

With this idea comes an awareness of a responsibility that I witness people swat away every day, as if it's not really there. This responsibility is difficult for some to swallow, as it engages you as the sole individual responsible for your every effort. It forces you away from your hiding place, from behind others' shadows, and out into the spotlight of the universe. With the essential, enlightening gifts that this presents to us for the positive, comes an irrefutably annoying reality check of realizing that we have to clean up our own messes. Rather than subtly using those in our life by depending on them for things we could easily provide for ourselves; instead of fudging the rules in our favor or looking to others to fix our problems, we find integrity at our feet, and choose to take full ownership over every aspect of our lives.

Ani may have said 'your body is your only true dominion', but our body is not nearly as important as *our* essence: our soul. Instead of choosing for your head or your body, choose, instead, to sit quiet with your heart and soul open before you. Choose to listen to their wisdoms, their hankerings, their desires: these are *your* most pure, most essential truths that you're gleaning! Taking the time to lower your defenses (yes, we even try to hide from ourselves), can open up a channel between you and your awareness; and between your essential truths, and your awareness. This, most hopefully, would take you to a moment where you receive everything you've ever desired. It would take time, and just as with any relationship, there would be communication backfires: sometimes we misunderstand our heart's desire, or we have a true moment of weakness and allow our ego to take the wheel for a second. But in the end, your perseverance to your higher self would reward you with life experiences and moments that extend beyond your absolute wildest dream.

It really sucks, to have to live without ego in order to experience a fulfilling, enriching life. I sometimes still wish to take the easy road, and get away with it. But there is a sense of universal justice (we could use the word karma, but we don't have to) present all around us that can really bring the hammer down, if you're not careful. I've played with Lady Justice' fire... and I shall do my very best to stay far away from her flickering snare for the rest of my time here, and on into the next. We may not always get to have all the experiences or opportunities that we so desire, but we really do only have so much time on earth. Do we want to waste it doing the things that 'everybody else does', or do we want to, instead, savour the flavours meant for our particular palate!?

The pressure of building your story

It can be difficult to break away from the people and things that you love and hold dear, especially when you are doing so for the sake of a more personally attuned reality. But you deserve to build what you seek. And you do not need to make yourself feel guilty or restrained for taking the time out of your life to cultivate and create this space that will benefit every aspect of your life positively, including the relationships with those reluctant to the changing winds a-blowin'. Regardless of others' initial timidities to the change, be bold; be the current of change that carries others to a new shore, more beautiful than any they've witnessed before!

I was once faced with a life-altering, impossible decision. Or, at least it felt impossible in the moment I had to make it. My mum was in the hospital, as the doctors had found a mass in her brain, and I was set to move to another state, halfway across the country, a week after we found out. Previous to this reveal, my mom had struggled a bit with some health problems, and for the longest time, I had been the one she depended on to help her live a more fulfilling life; I had been her confidant for so long, I could barely recall when it began. However, I have two older siblings, both of whom had moved forward in their lives by this point, and were starting families of their own... The tricky thing is, here I was all set to move out to another state to be with my significant other, but since we were just starting out, and my siblings had already manifested more cemented and well-established relationships, the responsibility to support my mum fell entirely to me, instead of to them.

Here I was, standing in the tiny hospital room of the NICU, surrounded by every person whom I was supposed to feel comfortable enough to depend on, but most of whom had been depending on me for years, as tangents to my mother, asking me to babysit, or to help with an overload of work, or to drive this person here, and drive that person there.... So anyway, there I was, watching twelve pairs of eyes stare back at me with the full, blatant expectation that it was obvious (to everybody except me) that I should be the chosen one to let go of their future to stay to help mom. I could not believe it. I could not believe my eyes! I was so shocked and amazed, to see how readily they were all willing to sacrifice my future for me, so they could preserve theirs. It woke me up to a very harsh - *very* difficult - pill to swallow about an objective surveyance of the majority of my life.

I finally saw a brilliant, bright truth my family had been dampening on a regular basis to help their own hides: that they used me, they did so on a regular basis, and they didn't mind. They had justified themselves out of the guilt too long ago to notice the shift. And just like that, my mind was clear. Well, first I had the biggest panic attack of my life, my brother had to walk me out of the building to get some air, but then it was all clear. I finally understood an essential truth I had been abiding by, while no one else was. I realized, from that experience, just how much I valued others' time, effort, and energy; and I also realized how much of a gap existed between how much I valued them, and how much they valued me. I had been used, by the very people who were supposed to stand by my side and prohibit anyone else from using me as they had been doing for such a long time.

Now, I of course postponed my move, and continued to be there for each of my family members as I had always done, just... less. I slowly backed away from the life I didn't want, that it was apparent I didn't want, but that apparently nobody cared enough to help me exit. I made peace with my decision, in knowing that I was barely surviving under the weight of their apathy for my existence, and that I was serving my higher purpose by still deciding to move, to be with an honorable man who valued the same ideals as I; a man who stuck up for me when I couldn't stand up for myself. Nowadays, my relationships with each of my family members are so much stronger than before, and are flourishing beautifully, because I chose happiness, and because I lived by my essential truths, while they lived by theirs. This is true peaceful coexistence! We are a happy, united family that now supports one another, communicates for their own needs, takes care of their own shitpiles, and doesn't judge or fearfully push around one another.

How to combat these pressures

Apply happiness to absolutely every situation, and it will flow your way like a river to the ocean. Use this as an essential ideal for all of life. If you choose to approach a situation with straight-up happiness, instead of angst, fear, contempt, anger, impatience, frustration, anxiety, or the like, more happiness with attract to you, and the complex emotions will fall by the wayside. 'But will I still feel things other than just happiness? It sounds boring and uneventful'. You may wonder, but only in vain, as the calmness of our own nature will fulfill us, in more ways than we can anticipate, and the daily dramatics of the past will be outed for their insignificance amidst what matters.

You choose your emotions. You can choose to rid yourself of the more complex emotions that cloud your view of the best pathway forward in any engagement. If you struggle with this, as I have, practice thinking about yourself less. Practice forgetting what you're feeling in a moment of strong emotion - try to simply release it, and let it leave your mind, so that you can refocus, with clarity, upon the truth of the matter at hand, whatever that matter may be. Just as you want to get down to the essence of your interests, objects, and whatnot, you want to pare down your more unnecessary emotions - or, the ones that cloud the clarity you can achieve - so as to relinquish so many of the things that plague your existence.

Are you often confused during conflicts? Do you walk out in the middle of a fight? Or, do you always get too emotional to communicate? As a former emotion addict, I have to vouch for the clearer side of things. Clearing out the unnecessary emotions will clean up your conflicts, allowing you to bypass the verklempt overwhelm of emotions in the face of conflict, to then communicate clearly and freely, listening without pride or angst, and responding without aggression or malice. Your relationships just got a whole lot better, my friend. Boom. The way to fix any problem is, of course, to start at the root. And the root of misfire in the face of conflict is an overwhelm, or a cluttering, of emotions. Once we clear that out of the way, we can walk into the face of any conflict, and communicate our thoughts, emotions, and perceptions with clarity and easy. Go away, miscommunication! You're not welcome anymore. We don't want no. Just like scrubs.

Once you clear away all that emotional clutter, rays of sunshine will shoot into your life, igniting any corners of darkness, and revealing opportunities previously unseen. They were there all along; only, you needed to shift your perspective to see them! Once you allow happiness to seep into the places of your life where it didn't exist previously, I guarantee that you will see more beautiful things surrounding you, than ever you noticed before! Additionally, you will be so much more grateful for what you *do* have than what you do not, and for who you *are*, rather than who you are not, that abundance and beauty will attract to you like a magnet! As I often mention, the Law of Attraction is something you can allow to work against you, or work with you to gain benefit from!

DETERMINING WORTH

How to determine what you really care about

In our world of... everything, how do we determine what has value; i.e., what really matters? Doing it all doesn't mean doing it well; and, the more you do, the less you have time for. The more 'filler' in your life, the more clutter you have to weed through to get to the good stuff. Choosing wisely what your essential wants and needs are, and applying your energy and attention thusly, will allow you to finally see the purpose, meaning, and direction of your life. As well as the steps to take to achieve your essential goals.

Instead of feeling as though you only ever make minimal progress in a million different directions, or that you are constantly exhausted from exerting a lot of energy - excess energy input, with no visible output - you can feel relief and peace away from the troubles that torment the worried and busy mind, if you apply these essentialism ideals into your life. In the buddhist practice, this sort of busy, scattered mind is called a "monkey mind', because of how scatteredly primal its thoughts and instincts are. This is how we have to be when we are multitasking, and then running from one thing to the next without end or pause: we have to survive the craziness that it truly is, and in order to do so, our minds have to exist, consistently, in a fight or flight mode, to an certain extent.

However, this chronic existence in fight or flight mode is not congruent to aptitude or excellence. In order to encourage our best, and be able to achieve our desires, we must remain mindfully aware of our surroundings, and give our best, with purity and integrity. Not with vulnerability and ignorance - these are attributes that cloud our clarity of perception; whereas, purity and integrity are more clean, pure emotions, free from so much excess or baggage.

In regards to physical traits or habits; i.e., things you wouldn't expect to be culprits of a lack of mindfulness, but that often are: we want to be aware of what we experience, feel, or witness, and especially so within ourselves. For example, I am very uncoordinated, in the sense that I often run into things, and often in odd places or unexpected ways. My arms always hit the side of doorframes as I walk through; my feet get caught on ridges and curbs tripping me up (or down, rather...);

and I always seem to hit my legs on the side of bed frames or couches or coffee tables as I pass by, regardless that I was convinced that I had had enough room to get through. I used to excuse these encounters as just a part of who I was, all set, never to change my ways, and to be bruised up for all eternity. However, now I see these as simple reminders, to stay present to the current moment. Each of these 'love taps' I receive, from the spaces I walk within, only stand to show and remind me to be mindful and attentive to all of my surroundings, and to the the people within them. As a result, I run into things less, and am more coordinated overall!

When we find ourselves at a crossroad, we often experience cognitive dissonance, or a mental discomfort caused by the intersection of two contradictory beliefs. This can cloud our minds on the daily, if we're unsure about who we are and what we desire. For example, I want to go on a hike, but I'm trying to spend less gas money; or, I want that cake, but I am gluten free now. These incongruencies of thought keep our minds so busy, that the decision making then takes up so, so much - way too much - of our time! If we choose, instead, to take the time to focus inward, and decide for ourselves what we truly value most in the world, we will acquire a freedom and clarity of mind that is incomparable!

How do you determine what you really care about? You ask yourself questions, and not just the easy ones. Dig deep. Instead of the curious pondering of what you would have and do if the options were limitless, consider your true nature. Consider the possibility that this switch could fulfill your heart's deepest desires better than anything you've ever known, and make everything in your life feel more lush, fulfilling, satisfying, enticing, emulsifying... I could go on. You will sense your life in beautiful, subtle ways that ignite a real, live passion in your belly, and you will find what you seek, as you are, then, living within your means, but without your limitations.

How to determine priorities

Am i investing my time and energy into the right things for my essential journey? Quick - somebody count how many times I use a variation of 'essential' within the book! If you want to feel a greater sense of fulfilment and worth, pairing down the amount of things you focus on can work wonders. Pick three things to focus on: one person, one thing, and one activity. Narrow it down to as minimal of a selection as you can; as specific and choice as you are capable of crafting. Then, focus on these three things, and only these three things. If, let's say, you want it (or need it) to be four or five things, rather than three, that's more than alright - this is for you, after all - however, I will dissuade you from picking too broad of elements. For example, choose to focus on cooking, rather than everything involving the kitchen, or choose to improve the intimacy of your relationship, rather than want for a supremely perfect relationship. Perhaps just focus on one element of an interaction you have with someone; or, on mastering a specific skill that would enhance your self-worth, as well as your journey, quite nicely.

Try to avoid letting things feel like they're ticked off a list once you complete them. You wouldn't want to make the accidental mistake of simply continuing to live for an obsession of 'getting things done'. Some of the busiest people I've met only end up running circles around the same patch of dirt their whole lives, and being exhausted the entire time. And not that this is bad, per se, but it is non-essentialist in mind. Consider what you truly want to accomplish in your life, and then assess whether you are taking the necessary steps to accomplish your essential goals.

The wisdom of innocence ignites a flame of understanding for us as adults; by connecting with our primordial self, we learn more about our essential nature. Most people hold true to about five or six main values, give or take, of course. True self-awareness unfolds like a lotus flower on our laps once we recognize the intrinsic values we hold to. This is where we apply a more selective criteria to what is truly essential to us, to then determine how much of ourselves we should put into each thing we do. Once we connect with our innate wisdoms and visions of ourselves, a whole heck of a lot of clarity arises. Whether you choose to live a pristinely minimal and essentialized life, or you gently tug some of these concepts into your journey very subtly, sorting out your essential values is invaluable, and essential to finding clarity in the everyday.

To figure out your top values, make a list of everything you think exists as a value. You can include such ideals as Adventure, Creativity, Balance, Integrity, Recognition, Loyalty, Wisdom, Wealth, Power, Health, Fame, Helpfulness, and Business Success. You define what the values are. You can even do some research into finding out what those who have written and publicly shared information about finding values define them as. Make sure that the final list is *your* engineering, and that it comprises only how you see the world, and what you see as values. Perception is everything, after all. Ensure, however, that you consider everything that influences your life, good and bad. Think about what brings you joy, causes you to fear, makes your uncomfortable or smile, makes you angry, humble, or whatever. Jot these down as possible values.

Once you've got your list, narrow it. As you would with anything, narrow it to a top ten. Then a top five, which is where your focus should remain. Then order these five from your most sacred to least. Now, you could rattle off your values anytime! Just, be sure to check back in with yourself as you grow and change, as our core values can fluctuate with us over time. Also, be sure that these values really are your core values, and not just the means to a sought-out end. For example, if you want financial independence because it will give you freedom, then what you *really* value is freedom, not finances. From the moment you discern your values and onward, you will find much more clarity around where your priorities lie. They align with your values! For example, my core values (at least, for the moment) are Universal Connectivity, Freedom, Intimacy, Wisdom, Pleasure, and Integrity. These align directly with my priorities: I always put my mindfulness, and connection to the universal energy, first. I won't leave the house unless I am not connected to myself, and am centered and grounded. Too much of life can surprise you, in the least suspecting of moments, and I prefer to be prepared with the support of the universe at my shoulders.

When to say yes and no

The pull of feeling busy and 'having a lot of friends' is strong. But as I mentioned before, it does not have to dominate your existence, like a rule book or strict schedule you have to follow. You do not owe anyone anything, so much as you deserve to give yourself the best existence; the best, most joyful and fulfilling journey you could ask for. And remember the freedom that can be found in setting boundaries for yourself, with the individuals in your life, and with the things you choose to focus on.

Say yes to the things that align with your values. For example, if I am trying to save money, I'm not going to choose to go to a store. I would be baiting disaster, already choosing outside my values, thus allowing for even more mishap to slip through the cracks. If your value is freedom, save up your money, and cut any emotional ties with those who make you feel like you are uncomfortable with yourself. Well, I guess I shouldn't say to just cut ties with them. Instead, always try to give it a go! I find that, sometimes, we are the ones who cage ourselves, yet we blame it on the other person, or people. At times, we are made to see something in ourselves that we don't want to see, because of the person, or people, we are with; due to something in their essence, that doesn't align with ours.. This allows us to presume that it is the other person's 'fault', when really it is only our own weakness; cowardice.

If you are tired of the struggle to 'barely keep up' with your friends, yet constantly feel busy without the showings of productivity, allow yourself to say no. Say no to parties, friends, family events, any of it. Don't go nuts, just… don't be too shy or modest. Make the time you need, for yourself. You must. If you want to stop feeling so overworked, yet underutilized; and like, perhaps, your time is often hijacked by others' agendas, you must remember that you decide. Guilt, fear, frustration, angst, loneliness… none of these emotions comfort us at night. They will only let you down, so leave them, and instead of always saying yes to others, say yes to yourself!

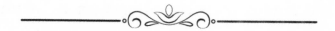

ACCOMPLISHING

How to do less and accomplish more

My siblings were successful immediately after school. They each started businesses that took off, wherein which they got to be creative, doing things they really loved with the majority of their time. I always looked up to them, and figured that it would end up with three out of three of the siblings finding easy successes. I was wrong, but not because I was not talented, or capable. Only, or at least mostly, because I was getting in my own way, limiting my own success, by figuring it to be a formula I could properly fill myself into. I imitated both of their 'every moves' combined, and added in some of the examples of my favorite idols. Soon enough, I was chasing my own tail with busyness... and going nowhere. Plus, I was spending so much of my time [all that lost time] *not* actually being myself. I spent all that time trying to climb the ladder of business success by acting like everybody else.

It wasn't until I took a bit of time away from my family, that I realized what I had been doing for so long. I saw, upon the separation, just how much I had been formulating myself to make others like me, or give me an advantage. No one ever told me that I came across rude or... anything of the sort, but I cringe now, whenever I look back on those times. And, what's more: as soon as I stopped trying to imitate my way to success, and began believing in myself fully, success actually started attracting itself to me! It was the darndest thing! It makes me feel like the universe wants us to truly be ourselves, and be good people, and will reward us for such! Even if it's untrue, I enjoy the idea, and consider it fondly.

The ideal of success can cloud our minds, distracting us from ever fully attaining the successes we set out to. Distractions distract. By zeroing in on what you desire to achieve, your mind will spend more effort, your energy will more efficiently exert, and the universal matter will attract to you more success, so long as you can believe it. These desires can, and most certainly should, align with your essential values. Only choose a handful of items upon which to focus, tops, so as not to spread yourself more broadly than is efficient or worthwhile in the long run.

Focus yourself on tasks that have value. In your life and work, you will be much better off, and get much further along, if you can focus your mind to completing those tasks first, without procrastination. How do you determine the tasks with the most value? You weigh out how they relate to your prime values. For example, I have to choose between doing the laundry, writing for a gig, organizing some gallery shipments, or writing a piece to submit for a prize. While I am most excited to write the piece for the competition, I need to choose wisely, with my best long-term interests in mind. I choose to organize the gallery shipments, as they are my primary source of income, and one of my main values is (financial) freedom. Then, I do the writing gig, so again I work towards that freedom. Next, I would do the laundry or write the competition submission. Perhaps, multitask… whatever! You don't need to be *so* utilitarian about your choices and their order, to such an extreme extent, if you don't want to. Just, try to put your value-based work first, then allow for the rest to follow after. Everything in its place; all things in balance.

How to antidote the stress and anxiety of what others are accomplishing

Rather than granting implicit permission to others, through submission, thus allowing them to take advantage of your time and energy, reclaim your control. Take back your choices; your decisions, and bask in their beauty. Take back the right to feel free from others' expectations, perceptions or unwarranted opinions. Take it all back, and hang out by yourself for a second. Feel what it feels like to be you, sitting still, without goals; without disappointments, fear, or anger; without vendettas or jealousy or pride; without any of this getting in the way, and, instead, joy, grace, and ease washing over you, supplying you with all that you need. You no longer need to be busy and constantly striving to 'have it all'. You supply yourself with 'it all', now, separate and outside of others' complaints, worries, issues, or comments.

I do not believe it is necessarily a bad thing if you become a bit of a loner for a short time. You have to leave the ring every once in awhile. And you sure as all cannot run anything on a battery that isn't charged. I find that the occasional, uncomfortable chunk of time spent in true solitude can really be beneficial to our true selves. It allows us to only feel our own energy; only breathe our own air, thus allowing our truest selves to slowly unfold like a lotus flower before us. When we do find ourselves sitting quietly with our true nature, we can ask ourselves things that are likely quite uncomfortable to sit with in our more exposed and vulnerable moments. This is precisely why we take time all by ourselves; so that we allow ourselves ample amount of time to release into the truth and wisdom we hold so tightly within our inner coils.

So, allow yourself this time. And if, for some reason, you doubt that it is worth taking time away from your busy, people-filled life to be alone, or that you cannot imagine telling others what you're up to if you do, just consider this an act of survival. You will, eventually, burn out from the exhaustion of your busy life; you absolutely have to recuperate and recharge; it's a need. And anyone who doubts that doesn't have the right to make your decisions for you, so do it anyway.

Why accomplish anything?

At times, I find myself not wanting to accomplish anything at all, and instead, just want to sit around, be lazy, and not care about anything - at all. However, then, after a moment of this (even if it's a long one), I want to *do something* again; be something; strive; attain. I want to build, grow, and expand in consciousness - this is our nature, as humans, as well as - in my opinion - somewhat of our duty. We crave adventure, experience and understanding. This constant and consistent growth process gives us comfort, in a very uncomfortable world. We yearn, even when we are balanced in yin and yang, and our ego is in check. We desire. So, we might as well fulfill what we desire, to as close of an experience as we dream about, as possible! We might as well accomplish our goals and dreams, especially if they are what makes us who we are; are our contribution to the world; and make the world grow in exciting, positive ways. This kind of momentum makes the whole world stronger, better, and a more positive place to exist.

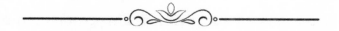

FULFILLMENT

Discipline Your Desires

The cost of trying to do it all is going nowhere. Doing a few things *really well* can build a very meaningful life; one that matters. Feeling fulfilled is different than feeling unique or important or funny or whatever. Fulfilment is the feeling of satisfaction that you glean from transforming the imagined into reality: by actualizing what you desire; by making your dreamiest of dreams come true. There are different levels of fulfilment, but the truest of all is the kind that sustains you. Just as there are levels of support in the food we consume, there are levels of fulfilment. In terms of food, you want to avoid the simple sugars that only leave you lonely and energy-less; instead you choose to consume the complex sugars that will take longer for your body to break down and, thus, supply your body with the energy it needs to sustain you for a much longer length of time.

If you are indecisive, or don't want to have to choose just one thing to focus on at a time, you're in danger of spreading your efforts so thin that you make absolutely no impact at all in the world around you. If you want to change course, and you want to make an impact, you have to act differently. Your only way out of the vicious cycle of discontent is to discipline yourself. You've found out what your values are, and now you must align everything you do to those values, in a prioritized and organized fashion. If your core values are freedom, intimacy and family, in that order, for instance: you wouldn't decide to go to a family function if it made you feel like you would lose your freedom, as that would be putting your primary values in harm for the sake of lesser ones. Or, at least, you would guard yourself carefully if you did attend. However, if your main value is spending quality family time, and you don't have a previous engagement, you would do whatever it took to attend the family event. See what I mean, here? Align your actions with your desires. This alignment will naturally encourage, then, an integrity of spirit that proves a useful and engaging support to all of your endeavors. Don't let yourself do whatever you want at every moment. Come up with a system for yourself, or find a mentality that works to help you stay true to the course. As soon as you first experience that thrill of true fulfilment, you won't want the quick fixes anymore, I guarantee you. And, if you do still want the quick fixes, that's ok - so do I! I just manage them a bit better than I used to, and don't give in so easily to my whims.

Further down this line is the idea that you don't ever just do whatever you want anymore, willy-nilly; at least, not if you want to fully embody and achieve what you desire. I'm sorry to say it, but you don't get to eat your cake, and ice cream, and tiramisu, and créme brulée. Wouldn't that be far too much to handle, anyway? I mean, as enjoyable as it is to pig out, the finesse of choosing wisely can allow for a much deeper, much more expansive joy to fill you up when you do indulge, and facilitate a state of being where you want for nothing for a little while. This is why trained monks can go without food or water: they have found deeper wisdoms and spiritual truths that fulfil them beyond want or need; they only consume to sustain. They cultivate their desires outside of instant gratification; in other words, they're playing the long game. That is, unless pigging out is your core value; then, feel free to pig on out and enjoy your life! Just, still, consider disciplining for the sake of longevity!

This disciplining of your desires can be the very thing you choose to focus on, all by itself. Maybe all you need to do is back off a little, and indulge a little less, overall. From the internet, to chocolate, to fried chicken (one of mine)... whatever it is you may have the tendency to overindulge in. You may come to find, upon considering this pairing down of interests, that your mind wanders to wonder, 'But won't I just stop caring about everything? If I start to care less about what others think? If I start to care less about how much "succeeding" I am accomplishing compared to others, won't I just be lazy and never accomplish anything?' No. No, you won't. This is a falsity. You will, most likely, just appreciate more of what you truly desire, rather than just more of everything. This will help you to feel more fulfilled, from less. You won't have to work so hard; you'll be confidently content in what you *do* have, versus distracted by what you don't.

Finding fulfilment (and sticking with it)

You have to pave the pathways to the adventures you wish to go on! You have to weed away the distractions from your life, in order to make the space necessary to explore the world around you. I never understood this, previous to my transformation into essentialism. I was adamant that if I didn't do everything now, as much and as perfectly as possible, my whole life would end up being for nothing, and I wouldn't matter at all. The thing is, though, that I don't have to do a *thing* for my life to be considered worthwhile; at least, I don't have to do anything for the sake of others' approval or attention. All I need to do is focus on what matters the most to me, because that is what will make me look back on my life and consider it one worth living.

At the end of the day, people really do come and go from your life; the natural ebb and flow of life draws some close, while sending others off. So, those we may choose to wrap our whole lives around potentially end up leaving us, thus leaving us without meaning or purpose... unless we truly are following our own desires. Following your desires doesn't mean you bypass pain and discomfort, however. These feelings initiate growth, and are important to us, in fulfilling our life's journey. Just, you can live a life with a lot less discomfort, pain, and suffering if you recognize yourself and your place in the world, and swim with the current of your life, rather than trying to swim upstream because it is someone else's current, and it looks prettier than yours. You're never going to get there, my friend. You're going to die trying, and you're going to be miserable and unhappy the entire time. Why make yourself miserable and unhappy just so you attain others' love and approval?

Also, age. You do not need to be of a certain age to attain certain wisdoms, or have certain dreams fulfilled. The dream of the nineties may be alive in Portland, but the dream of the fifties is dead as a doorknob, and no one remembers where it was buried, anyways. It's probably in one of the thousands of time capsules that no one will ever dig up, scattered somewhere in the American soil beneath us. You are meant to soar above those who raise you and try to teach you; your insight and pursuit can carry you anywhere you dream. We all learn, see, experience, and incorporate differently with the space around us. Don't wait for anything: to grow up, to be respected, to be admired. Nope! Make it happen, if you want it. You need not prove or pay any dues in this world, except to respect the earth, and remain steady on your quest for your own, personal higher truth.

There is a status symbol attached to action, and most especially, to the proof of the action, in the current world. We are made to think that we only 'matter' when we do cool stuff, and showcase or broadcast it to the world around us. I feel these tides slowly changing, however; what once was essential to perceived success in America will deplete itself of its energy. This obsession with curating our life for all the world to see, as though we only live our lives for the sole feedback and perceptions of others; as though those around us are our bumpers, keeping us on the straight and narrow of what is most beloved and accepted by the masses, is at a close. Soon, we will start keeping our secrets sacred again.

Now that everything has been blast into the spotlight, individuals will start to feel uncomfortable on the stage, and prefer to hang back in the shadows, instead. You might as well get a running start on the currents of change, by choosing to recognize this, and act as such. You may as well start to see how much your actions' relevancy is not in correlation with public acclaim. You need not broadcast or showcase your life. You are worthy of love, from others and yourself. In order to feel the love, truly in your bones, recognize yourself as worthy, without any conditions. You deserve to feel the support of unconditional love from those in your life, as we all do. In the world of the moment, it can be hard to know where to go for truly deep connection; where to search for intimacy. There are so many illusions and liars abound, and especially so when they can so easily hide behind a computer, phone, or tv screen. Don't just trust screens blindly, ever; they are illusions, and while some truth filters through, there exists a whole hell of a lot of impurities and deceit that come along with it.

Break away from the chains that bind you to convention. Live I've said, you do not need to experience what others experience. You don't need the same clothes and makeup; don't need to shop at the same stores. You don't need to go to the same events, games, or see the same performances. You just need to do you, and do so with confidence and edge. By golly, if enigmas aren't the most fascinating things on earth! I've fancied myself an enigma, ever since someone told me, "boy, you are quite the enigma" in college. I've always somewhat prided myself on that moment, as I had, since forever, held an austere reverence for mystery. There's something so beautiful about mystery; something so curious; so educational. You are curious and original, at your core, and need not pretend to be anything but. Be an enigma. Shock others. Be the person who surprises people with how they engage with the world, if that's what it means to truly be you. Don't fall into the same patterns and mechanisms; mentalities and opinions, as those surrounding you. Question the world, and let it know you want to know its secrets; its truths.

Choose to see past the ignorance and pride that we cover ourselves in; these sheaths of emotional armor that protect the delicacy of true intimacy. Go deeper in. Into yourself, into the world. And then: expand your mind. Move past the options that tv dramas, magazines, media, and others' opinions present to us as a populace, and see the subtle, gorgeous, glowing orbs of wisdom that sit behind all the illusions, amidst the subtle realms of expression. See past the whole to the individual. Choose to allow your creativity to flow to every aspect of your life like lava: from the products you use and how they're made, to the kind of content you choose to allow the media to feed you, to your health and wellbeing, and even to how you fix objects. See that there are more possibilities than the solutions laid out by professionals. These professionals have narrowed their focus so much, that all they know is what they have to work with, and what they are paid to push. Push past this idea that professionals know best, or that they have it all figured out, and that there's no other options. It's simply not true! True evolution occurs when the things we seal as 'finished', or figured out, are put into question. Is the world round? Maybe, but many people out there believe that it is not, and, someday, one of them may just be the next Einstein or whatever, and prove it to the world that we live in an orb, or something, and that we've always thought the earth was round because of a reflection... or something. I'm riffing, here, so go easy! [This is where, in a text or an email, I would generally insert a winky face emoji.]

NATURAL BALANCE

The Balance of Nature; The Balance of our Lives

We've all heard the saying, "It's the journey, not the destination." This couldn't be more true, but I don't know about you, I just never seem to really give a shit about idioms like that. They mean absolutely nothing to you until you experience something that makes you fully comprehend and understand its meaning. But this is one of the truly amazing aspects of life, is it not? We can go through our entire lives without understanding a certain, particular kind of wisdom that another individual may have mastered day one. It all depends on our journey, and what we experience, struggle with, overcome, work through, and stand to handle. Charles Bukowski, a favorite poet of mine, wrote: "What matters most is how well you walk through the fire." If this weren't more true! And again, I didn't fully understand this until I was standing amidst the flames, but oh well! That is the beauty of life, is it not? Is that not what

Bukowski is on about? The beauty is in the struggle; in the discovery of a new insight.

Once you take the space you need, from the aspects of your life, everything will sort of settle into place, resetting the balance of the energies. Our lives want to be balanced; every yin craves its yang, and vice-versa. We all crave this kind of balance around us. And the way it works is, once you change, the world will change to meet you; once you shift, the world will shift with you. Whether this is because we manifest our realities, or because we attract ourselves to what we desire, you will most likely notice that it's not so much the elements of your life that change, than it is the way in which you've been seeing and perceiving the elements of your life that makes a causal shift. Suddenly, everything has more of a clarity of intention, purpose, and meaning, allowing us the space to feel grateful for what we have. Space allows is clarity of perception; discernment of emotion, and allows us to realize the freedom we have from our attachments. It can be the most blinding thing of all, feeling strongly about things to allow them to overtake your clarity. There's this other Ani DiFranco line, from her song *Garden of Simple*, where she says, "and, you know, they never really owned you / you just carried them around / and then one day you put 'em down / and found your hands were free." Now, obviously we all know that Ani DiFranco was a big part of my musical and poetic development, when I bring her up twice within one book, but that's beside the point. The point is, that the things that you think control you and make the rules up for you, are only convincing you of their prominence, by attempting to lure you to exert more energy in their direction. Just don't do it! Do the opposite of Nike! Don't do it, and, instead, put those things down; find that you're truly free so long as you choose to be.

Meaningful Clarity

When one decision makes a thousand at once, you will find clarity. Assimilating your values into your life will offer you a sense of freedom that remains unmatched. Don't you desire a fresh sense of awareness toward all that surround you? I'm sure that you, much like myself, can see the places in your own life where tension, frustration, anger, or general foggy emotions have built up, perhaps building with them some very real tensions that we don't want to have to face. But, by simply taking a step out of our day to day, we initiate and create the space for change to just occur, without much effort from us. In fact, if anything, we have to make sure that we don't get too involved or get in the way enough to mess things up. Once we allow the time and space for clarity to seep into those foggy or confusing places, there may still be tension, but it will look much less scary, and will be half as intimidating, or less. We can, then, tackle our fears with fresh perspective, a clear and acute perception, and a stabilized, focused, and determined mind.

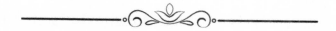

FOCUS

How to focus on the right things

Accepting the negative side of essentialism is (1) essential to your complete understanding of the concept, and (2) important to your choosing and embodiment of the accurate essentials for your personality. You have to know the positive and negative; the yin and the yang of any good thing.

Being able to accept the consequences of having less will force you to put more pressure; more focus, on what you *do* have. Because you have less to focus on, you are forced to put more expectation on yourself in a very delicate way. You don't want to put expectations on yourself in the sense that you set unrealistic and unattainable goals for yourself on daily basis. This is imbalance, and we are searching for balance. In this balance, you focus on the right things, expect yourself to embody what you are capable of with integrity, and follow through with joy and grace balancing your heart.

Once you choose to choose less and focus more, each and every thing in your life, and in who you are, is expected to be more; to do more. More, while being less. You put more pressure on yourself to deliver the deliverable, rather than hop scotch around from thing to thing, without any structure, integrity, or balance in mind.

I am a budding herbalist of sorts, and have taken various online classes to learn about all sorts of natural healing techniques. I believe very strongly in being the ambassador for your own journey, in every respect, including health. Doctors see so many cases and patients, that they know how to address symptoms, not people. They understand, in a mathematical and somewhat linear way, how to heal their patients. However, healing is *not*, by any means, linear and mathematical in nature. Nor does it just occur on a physical level. Healing is a multitudinous and faceted experience of obtaining wisdom and exploring ourselves in new ways in order to cultivate and grow in new directions. Doctors do not know you. This is why only you can be the advocate for your own health journey. When healing occurs, it affects every level of the human existence, including energetic, physical, emotional, and spiritual. It is my belief that most, if not all, dis-ease begins on a vibrational level, or an emotional level. Dis-ease always begins with an imbalance in the system of some sort, and not always of the sort the doctor can heal. They may be able to treat the symptoms a thousand times over, but if you don't pull a weed up from its roots, it'll rear its ugly head forever.

You must be the advocate for your own human experience, and in order to do so, you've got to pay attention to yourself. I have struggled with digestion issues and food allergies my entire life, but until I combatted my anxiety, they persisted no matter what I tried. Once I recognized how linked my mind and stomach were, I understood how to heal. The healing was a long journey, and it took place through many peaks, valleys, and an ocean or two of tears. But now that I am on the other side of that journey, I am so much more joyful and at peace with the universe. Healing yourself heals the world - we are all connected, and every step you take towards the light, and away from the dark, brings the world one step closer to its emotional evolution.

Speaking of herbalism, when I first began to learn the craft, I was a bit overzealous with my online herb class shopping, and ended up with three cupboards full of every herb out there - or, rather, every herb the course recommended. I would go to the cupboards to pull out certain herbs and use them, get to know them... but a few years later, there were still herbs I hadn't ever gotten to, and while I hadn't gotten to them, their shelf life passed by in a flash. The herbalists I had been taking these courses from recommended that an early trainee spend a whole moon cycle, or about a month, with each plant, so they can connect with the plant not only on a scientific and informative level, but on a spiritual, emotional, and personal level, as well. Now, did I do this? No, no, of course I didn't. Had I refrained from purchasing so many herbs out of sheer, bumbling excitement, and had I paired down my focus as the herbalists had suggested, I may have gotten to know less herbs, yes, but I would have gotten to know the ones I focused on much, much better: their massages would be inked on my skin in recipes, applications, and benefits... rather than my still sometimes confused approach toward particular herbs, wherever the learning flow was stifled by the overflow of information I was trying to absorb all at once, at the time.

How to avoid the constant distractions / remove obstacles

I cannot drink very much caffeine. As soon as I've had more than I should, things start to hum and vibrate before me, and I move, in my words and in my physicalities, like a roadrunner on coke. Not that I've ever tried the stuff - I figure it would destroy me. Caffeine and sugar already do enough damage to my nervous system and adrenals, as it is. But anyways, too much caffeine makes me unable to focus for much too long. It ruins my productivity, and I quite honestly think I am really, pretty annoying when I get all amped up like that. I start speaking a million miles a minute, Gilmore Girls style, and can't slow up unless I take a natural, medicinal depressant. It's a travesty to encounter, to be honest, so I have to pay close attention as to when to stop drinking, whenever I decide to order one of those amazing, flavored latte concoctions.

This feeling of being revved up, and how I act when I am such, shows me a sped-up version of what I am already like, naturally, in the everyday. Which is why I have always firmly believed that we should not just be excused entirely for our actions when under the influence of a substance - substances simply present more dramatic, or played out, versions of ourselves, in some manner or another. When I take the time to notice the effects of a substance such as caffeine, and take note of how scattered and annoying I can be under its influence, I am able to see how those patterns run like rivers through me constantly. I, even still, struggle with making decisions, though I have my ego in check, and do not allow it to distract me with its instinctual, ego-filled desires. If I chose to simply hop around, from one unfinished project to the next, even if it were out of pure excitement, I would never have anything to show for my life - not really, except for a bunch of attempts and experiments, never fully followed through.

The hyper-connectivity of our current social landscape makes us feel like 'doing it all' is more possible than ever, but this is an illusion of the mind. Just because something *appears* to be more tangible, doesn't mean that it is. The internet does illusions better than most. It can easily convince us to reach for everything, in every possible direction. However, this leaves us limbless, and without a core to come back to; to depend upon. Thus, by following your values, you don't just go reaching for every apple that looks good; you decipher and decode your true essence, to come to a well-discerned decision on an aspect of your life.

Now, how else can we avoid the trappings of the overloaded life? Avoiding opinion overload. Opinion overload leads to information overload, which causes strain on our brains. We are so obsessed with what everyone else is doing, or with what everyone else thinks about what *we're* doing, that all we find ourselves actually *doing,* is trying to play catch up with those doing the *actual* doing. Make sense? By just filling your life up to the brim with people, things, events, ideas, and interests, there's barely any room for creation of cultivation in any one space or direction. There *is* no space or direction. Thus, everything is underdeveloped, or semi-developed, and few real results are seen.

How to avoid the chaos but still feel involved

I find routine to be freeing and opportunistic. Sure, I used to loathe and dread routine with every fiber of my being and wish it were dead and buried somewhere far away from me, but now, I find it stimulating and releasing to exist within a daily routine. You'll notice I consciously avoid the word 'schedule', as it has many negative connotations I would much rather avoid having to sort through. By applying this discipline for discerning what I desire, and only focusing on the right things, I so we can make the highest possible contribution towards the things that really matter.

Once you open up the space in your life, and choose to focus on a few still objects amongst the whirlwind of chaotic movement, you will finally be able to see the path open up before you, and you will be able to make the climb, to reach for your potential. And, ultimately, make a contribution of more substance and worth than you ever could have before, when you were spinning in circles, but staying in one place.

CONCLUSION

Do less, better

This is a whole new life you're trying out, now. Everything that you *have* known or been or done, is gone, and now it's just you in this moment, deciding. So: stripped away version of yourself... what do you want? Now that you've come to recognize your core values, what will you focus on? What will you commit yourself to, to benefit from, and sustain your joy upon?

Whatever it is, sit and sink into the appreciation of your own joyful existence; of your own meaningful choices.

By scaling back our focus to the vital few, we allow ample space for our pursuit towards success, and cultivate a fertile foundation upon which our creations flourish with ease! Just as you don't want to overcrowd plants in a pot, you don't want to overload yourself; otherwise, you will be suffocating your creativity, and your true nature. And for what? For the sake of saying you 'did it all'? More is not more, it's just... extra. 'More' is a constant disappointment, as you find yourself always reaching short of your true goals. And in this way, more is, in fact, much less.

So do less! But do it better. Focus on the things that make your heart sing, follow through on them, and then release your stronghold to the universe, for it to carry onward. Remember how your emotions attract themselves, and how, by filling your heart up with joy when you embody the things you decide to do, you will attract unfathomable amounts of joy back in your direction!

Be more, more easily

The more we do, the more exhausted we are. We just cannot keep up with all the responsibilities, so our mental and physical stress take the toll, causing imbalances and confusion left and right. When you are constantly shifting yourself around, almost morphing yourself just to complete every task as quickly as you can to accomplish them all, are you even living? There are very stark differences between accomplishing tasks, and accomplishing desires. Differences we must choose to be perceptive of, if we want to ever feel alive. How can you be alive, if you can't be perceptive? And, what's more, who are you? How can you know for sure who you are, when you go bumper-car-ing through life, allowing it to push you around at its leisure. I say we all take the power back. We need not succumb to the weakness of external pressures to be and do everything. We have the right, as individuals, to stand up for ourselves, and say no to the inane distractions that try to keep us immobile.

When you are seen and heard just a little bit less in your life, your voice holds more power. Like a dam that holds the water from flowing over. When you give it all away, you're burnt out, empty, everyone can see it, and no one cares to change it for you. You, alone, can stand up for yourself, and declare yourself no longer a slave to to-do lists, social responsibilities, or professional pressures of success. You, alone, decide whether you will commit to discerning your essential values, and disciplining your desires. And you, alone, choose whether you stay the course, and make your way toward the embodiment and fulfilment of your heart's deepest desires. By choosing less, you achieve more, and are able to make the most out of your time on earth; out of your existence. Once you know what gives your life real meaning, go after it, don't look back, and don't get distracted, because you can achieve whatever it is, so long as you are properly prepared for the journey, and are focused like a camera with impeccable zoom.

ABOUT THE AUTHOR

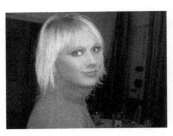 Aoife lives in the mountainous terrain of Colorado with her husband, and two dogs. She runs a small art gallery that focuses on living resources, especially when those are reclaimed, recycled, or reused. Aoife spends much of her time walking the Colorado terrain with her pups, playing the dulcimer in the mountains, and writing short fantasy and sci-fi stories, if only to indulge her own over-active, imaginative mind! She dreams of Scottish Castles and nights at sea, having long-winded conversations with Mother Nature.

Thank you for taking time to read *Essentialism* If you enjoyed it, please consider telling your friends or posting a short review.

Word of mouth is an author's best friend and much appreciated.

OTHER BOOKS BY AOIFE LEIGH CLARK

Declutter Your Mind

The Art Of Decluttering And Organizing Your Life...

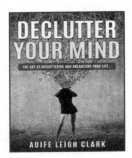

How to Win Friends

...and attract fulfilling relationships into our lives

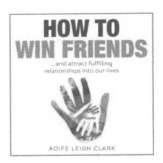

CPSIA information can be obtained
at www.ICGtesting.com
Printed in the USA
LVHW111605240720
661451LV00003B/347